# SUDDENLY SOLO
## *ENHANCED:*

### 12 STEPS TO ACHIEVING YOUR OWN TOTALLY INDEPENDENT HEALTH CARE PRACTICE

RICHARD A SCHOOR MD

*Dedicated to Robert S Schoor DDS*

*2-10-1935 to 11-17-2012*

*My Dad*

*My best teacher*

*I miss you, Padre, every day.*

# FORWARD

7 years ago, the greatest thing happened to me. I got canned. Sacked. Fired. Told to get lost. Kindly asked to not let the door hit me in the ass on the way out. I found myself suddenly solo. I was thirty-eight years old. I had a wife and two kids, and another on the way. I remember the experience like it was yesterday. It was painful, scary, and humiliating.

And liberating.

Yes, liberating. Contrast the liberation I felt then to the emotion I had several months earlier, before I got the boot, when I had hit a an epiphany of sorts in my career. On that day I stood in the office, which was actually a beautiful office and I looked at my surroundings; to my left, to my right, to my coworkers and partners working the factory floor, and I said to myself "my God, is this what I struggled for all these years? Is this it? Is this where I will spend the next thirty-five years of my life?" I felt my chest tighten and my throat close. I was suffocating. Is this despair? Fortunately three months later,

I was shown the door. Many people are not so lucky, and they remain in dead end, miserable jobs for decades. I certainly do not suggest that job loss is a good thing. For most people, job loss is among the worst of things that can happen during a lifetime. But for the right person, with the right skill set and right frame of mind, job loss can mean freedom. Perhaps you are that person.

In the introduction to my first edition of *Suddenly Solo: A Physician's Guide to Surviving and Thriving in Your Own Medical Practice*, I wrote that several hours after I was rendered suddenly solo, I awoke in the middle of the night with a sense of happiness—elation, really—that I had not had in years: the first of many "sleepless nights of endless possibilities and entrepreneurial dreams." Well, you know what? After seven years, I still feel that way. I still dream of the possibilities. I am happy.

This edition of my book, *Suddenly Solo Enhanced*, has been completely rewritten. The content is entirely original, updated, and has never before been published. Using feedback from the thousands of my blog readers and from the readers of the first edition of *Suddenly Solo*, I have made many changes; I think you'll find it a much-improved resource.

The book is not intended to be an all-encompassing guide to medical practice management or medical economics, nor is it intended to be textbookish. The book is intended to be a rough, down and dirty, and occasionally irreverent guide to professional practice start-up that can help you get out of a jam quickly, efficiently, and affordably. The lessons work best for the healthcare related fields but are also transferable to any professional service business. If you read the book, find it useful, and from it find hope and inspiration, then I have done my job. Conversely, if upon reading the book you determine that perhaps solo practice is not for you, then I have done my job as well; for when it comes to starting a solo practice, the time to quit is either before you start or after you have achieved success, but not in the middle.

One more thing—while this book certainly has a medical bent, most of the concepts apply to any professional service business. You can just pick and choose what applies to your specific profession.

With that being said, I now present to you *Suddenly Solo Enhanced: Twelve Steps to Achieving Your Own Totally Independent ~~Medical~~ (Health Care) Practice.*

# INTRODUCTION:

Why would someone, anyone, in this day and age open up his or her own health care practice? You'd have to be out of your mind to do that. Nuts! Solo practice in the United States is under full frontal assault. Increased governmental regulations coupled with bargain basement insurance reimbursements followed by decreased purchase power of all but the 1% of Americans has culminated in perhaps the worst time in the history of the US to be a solo doctor. So you'd think someone would need to have his or her head examined for going solo. That may be true, but for many of us who have tried group practice or academia or both, independent and solo practice was the only way that we could find happiness in medicine. And for others, still, solo practice was thrust upon us via a boot in our rear-ends. Personally, while I went into medicine in the first place to be my own boss, the catalyst for me was job loss; same for many others. How about you?

*   *   *

Imagine this: you are heading out the door at the end of office hours one Friday afternoon when you are summoned to the administrator's office and told that your continued presence at the medical/accounting/law practice will no longer be welcomed. WTF? You've been fired is WTF. No need to worry about your personal belongings, the administrator says, they will be sent by courier to your home.

Or try this one on for size. You show up to work one day to find that a guard blocks your entry into the office and seizes your ID badge from around your neck.

Personally, I like this one. You go away to a conference and when you return, you find that your current partners have decided behind your back that they no longer wish to work with you, and in your absence, they moved into *their* new location and took all the client records with them. Impossible, you say? Nope. Happened to someone I know.

Here's another dream scenario. You are going along at work, minding your own business and seeing patients, when you are introduced to your future replacement. I kid you not. Happened to another person I know.

This one could be humorous, so long as it happens to someone else: a physician at an academic institution gets called in for a meeting with his chairman. In a friendly sort of way, the chairman asks the doctor if anything is bothering him. The doctor speaks his mind honestly, and this honesty is rewarded with a boot in his rear end.

Job loss happens, and can threaten anyone; doctors, accountants, and lawyers are no exception. Think you are safe as a partner in your law firm or medical practice? Think again. Partner firings at law firms are on the rise; same with accounting practices. In fact, I believe that the risk of job loss to physicians, in particular, will actually increase in the coming years, as the contracts between the doctors and their hospital employer-masters expire.

Think it won't happen to you? Okay. Good for you. Stay in la-la-land. But if you believe that gravity affects you too, then start planning.

# WHEN SHOULD YOU START PLANNING YOUR EXIT?

---

Many of us, I included, ignore the signs that things are not going well in our current jobs, and plod along until the day the guillotine drops. Only then do we spring into action. Unfortunately, after the fact, in the face of the panic and humiliation of job loss, planning your next phase of professional life is too difficult. So when is the best time to plan for a career in solo, independent medical/professional service practice?

While it may never be too early or too late, in reality the best time to plan your exit is after you take your first job but while things are going relatively well. It is during this time that you should observe the operations of the practice. This way, you can learn on their dime, rather than your own. Befriend the secretaries, the medical assistants, the schedulers, billers, and surgical bookers, and pump them tactfully for information. See what kind of software the practice uses. Do they outsource their billing and if so, to whom, and do they like it? Talk to the partners and try to assess if they involve themselves in practice management, or if they seem more concerned with wine collecting or home decorating than they do with practice management. Finally get to know the office manager on friendly terms. Try not to make it so obvious that you want to learn practice management, just in case you get fired; but in reality, most practice managers would be thrilled to take someone under their wing. Even if word got out to the partners that you had an unusual interest in practice management, they would not likely hold it against you. Finally if you sense that things are not going your way—and you will know—for heaven's sake don't buy a house and get into major debt.

# THE TRUE STORY OF...

⸻

*The True Story of Dr. J*

*Dr. J, a fifty-year-old single mother, was an employed physician in a hospital-owned subspecialty practice. She worked hard, and her patients liked her. She even picked up a couple of her own good, referring doctors. As someone who had been in other practices prior to this one, she knew how things were done elsewhere, and she had good ideas. Unfortunately for her, the senior management team not only ignored her suggestions, they told her to keep her mouth shut and do what she was told. See, in this practice, Dr. J said, the management team cared primarily about RVU generation\*, to which their compensation packages were closely tied. Since she was salaried, she had no concerns herself over RVUs, and in fact, only had a vague idea of what an RVU was. As a result, her suggestions for improvements in patient care were ignored, unless they resulted in enhanced RVU productivity. Frustrated, she began to butt heads with management. Things were not going well for Dr. J at this practice. So what did she do?*

---

\* See appendix 1 for a discussion of RVUs.

*The only sensible thing—she bought a house with a big mortgage. Shortly after closing on her house, management informed Dr. J that her contract would not be renewed. At the same time, the group hired some young gun right out of training. Her replacement, perhaps? Management assured Dr. J that one thing had nothing to do with the other, and that she could stay for at least another six months. Her job was safe, she convinced herself. After all, she was loved by her patients and referring doctors. Surprise, surprise—she was axed a month or so into her new, six-month contract. Now she has a house with a big mortgage, a kid about to start college, and no savings.*

## The True Story of Dr. O

*Dr. O, a general surgeon, was an employed physician on a partnership track. The practice he joined was a great practice: very profitable and the partners owned both the surgery center, at which he operated, and a diagnostic laboratory. The partners seemed to have their hands into everything and the economic opportunities seemed great to Dr. O when he signed on with the group two years earlier. Initially things were swell; he was happy with the practice; and the practice appeared to be happy with him. Things only began to head south when Dr. O pushed for the partnership he was promised. The partners and administrators would yes him to death, but nothing ever happened. When push came to shove, he was repeatedly denied access to the practice's financial documents or his* own billing records. He must have pushed a little too hard, because one Sunday evening an administrator called him and told him not to come to work the next day. He was fired over the phone. Shock and humiliation turned to severe anxiety. Fortunately he had some money saved up and some entrepreneurial spirit. He did some homework, made a plan, and stuck to it. One year later he was self-sufficient in his own practice; bruised, but not destroyed. What does not kill you makes you stronger, they say, and after his ordeal, Dr. O is one strong mo-fo.

*The True Story of Dr. R*

Dr. R got what seemed to be a plum of a job right out of training. He was the envy of his co-residents. Things were looking good for Dr. R, and in July he packed his apartment and got into his Honda Accord and drove cross-country to start his new life. Dr. R arrived at his new office with a newly starched shirt and supreme self-confidence. He approached the front desk to announce that he had arrived; he was promptly given a clipboard and asked to sign in; and to furnish his insurance ID card. "I am sorry," he said. "You must be mistaken, as I am the new doctor the practice hired." Several minutes later the administrator walked out and Dr. R re-explained the situation. "Well, no one told me anything about this," she said. "Just sit here." It took an hour to clear up the mess and another couple days to find an office, a medical assistant, and clinic hours for Dr. R. Over the next two years,

*Dr. R consistently struggled for basic things like OR time, equipment, even a desk at which to sit. Dr. R did not make a mistake in joining this group. The group deceived him. He did make the mistake of buying a house, even though he knew that things were not going well for him professionally and that his time in this practice was very limited. But there was a silver lining to this story. Knowing that his time at this practice was limited, Dr. R was a sponge and learned what to do—and what not to do—in order to be a successful, independent doctor. He has made good use of that knowledge in his future endeavors, and continues to thrive today in his own medical practice.*

# STEP 1:

# DETERMINE YOUR PERSONAL FINANCES

———— ❖ ————

Building any business from scratch is difficult and expensive, and it can take years. Medical and other professional service practices are no exceptions. Before you commit to starting solo practice, it is imperative that you do an honest assessment of your own financial situation so that you can determine if the endeavor has even the potential to be a viable one. Do you have a working spouse, or are you the sole breadwinner? Do you have a too-large mortgage? Do you have credit card debt? Student loans? Child support? Are your kids about to start college? Can you afford health insurance? What are your costs of living?

Really take an honest look at your personal costs. Perhaps you may just need to find another job, at least temporarily, or maybe now is as good a time as any to strike out on your own. Only you can say. But you must be truly honest with yourself, unemotional and businesslike. Just because you want to go solo does not mean you can. After you figure out what you need personally to survive and whether or not you can meet those needs, only then you can proceed to step two.

The easiest way to determine our personal finances is to download 2-3 months of bank statements and to scrutinize them. Then do the same with your credit card statements. Look at where you and on what types of things, you spend your money; mortgage, groceries, cable TV, hair care, consumer spending, student loans, etc. Some things you can cut down or cut out, others you can't. You'd be surprised about how much you can ratchet down spending in times of need. On other hand, some people have overwhelming & suffocating debt. If that is you, then perhaps getting a job is the next step. Otherwise, proceed to the next step.

# STEP 2:

# MAKE A BUSINESS PLAN

---

When it comes to costs of doing business, not all professional service businesses are created equal. Medical practice, in comparison to virtually any other type of professional service business, is extremely expensive, and as a solo practitioner, 100 percent of those expenses fall on you. Therefore, before you commit to these professional/business overhead expenses, you must determine whether or not you will be able to meet them. Do you even have a sense of what the costs will be? Start by listing everything that you will need to be operational. List them on paper with a pen. You can find many examples of business plans in books or even online. You can purchase business plan software. You can go to business school. But the goal of your business plan is not to get an A from the business school professor, and you do not want to lose momentum because you are fretting over the "correct" way to make a business plan. Yet having a business plan is critical to the success of your venture, and it absolutely must be done. I simply cannot emphasize this enough.

Here is how I did mine. I took a piece of paper and listed on the left hand side all the things I thought I might need for my start-up. I listed everything: office, furniture, gauze pads, phones, insurance, equipment, financing, and so forth. On the right hand side I listed the strategies that I might employ to achieve my needs/goals. I revised my list at least a dozen times. Your list will not be complete either, and you will need to revise it over and over again, but that is okay. Just sit there and brainstorm the things you need and strategies to achieve them and their costs. After you have compiled your list, consult with someone who has been there before you, or someone who knows the medical business well, like a retired practice administrator. Alternatively you may simply take whatever costs you figured out and multiply them by a factor of two (or even four!).

It is during this step that you start to study the business of medical practice—or whatever your industry is. I read voraciously during this period (and continue to do so even now). Not only did I read about how to start a medical practice, I read everything I could get my hands on regarding small business in general; from dentistry, to accounting, to the pizza & hair salon businesses. I also talked to everybody and asked them how they did things. I actually got a pretty good pearl of wisdom from my local fishmonger.

You have a lot to learn, and one major problem is that you don't know what you don't know. Are you even aware of things like labor laws, statutory insurances, fire safety, payroll, FICA, cash flow, privacy laws and on and on and on infinitum? If you choose to go solo, you will need to deal with these things, even if you don't know about them.

There is one more thing. You really need 2 business plans: the short term one that gets you past the embryonic phase of business start-up and another long-term plan the gets you to where you want to be in 5, 10, or 20 years. In order to have a long term business plan you must have a guiding vision, an ultimate purpose, a dream practice—the one you always wanted but never thought you could have. Think big. Be audacious. You don't just want to be a dentist, you want to 90% implant dentistry to finance your passion of correcting congenital deformities in the 3rd world. You don't want to be just a family practitioner, you want to own 30 centers that help lower income Americans get quality health care.

The guiding vision allows you to stay the course as your practice grows and prevents you from making mistakes that take the practice in the wrong direction. For example, if you ultimate dream is to have a top-end plastic surgery practice, then perhaps contracting with a burn center might not fit with that goal and could take you off course. Early on in my new practice—when I was really hurting for money—a local nursing home wanted me to make rounds for them and see their patients. I declined their offer as it did not fit with my long term, guiding vision of developing a top-notch male infertility treatment center. At this point you may be struggling with the enormity of the short-term but the long-term plan is equally, if not more important.

Don't have a guiding vision? Get one. Just want to be a run of the mill doc (also called a commodity), then you may want to re-think the plan to go solo. But if you still think you can succeed, then proceed to step three.

# STEP 3:

# INCORPORATE

———————

A t this point, if you still think that you have a chance at succeeding long term in your new venture, you may want to consider incorporation of your new practice. As a medical doctor, your best options are one of two types: the limited liability corporation, LLC, or the professional corporation, the PC. You could remain unincorporated, which is called sole proprietorship. The only advantage of sole proprietorship is cost. It costs nothing. Sole proprietorship also affords you nothing in the protections that the law gives to corporations. Such protections include liability exposure and tax advantages, among others. For example, if an employee sues you over a labor dispute, or if someone falls in your office, or a creditor goes after you for non-payment of a lease, they can only go after the assets of the corporation. Your personal assets are protected.[1] You may come to rely on some of these protections in the future, so for this reason I recommend incorporation at this stage.

While there are low-cost, online methods to incorporate, I recommend using a lawyer to do it for your practice, so that it is done correctly. This will cost you about $1,000. If this is too much for you to pay then you may want to rethink your plan to go solo. If not, then proceed to the next step.

---

1  *Whether or not your personal assets are protected depends on a number of factors in addition to incorporation, such as terms of lease and personal guarantees on loans, rent, and so forth.

# STEP 4:

# GET A PHONE NUMBER

———— ••• ————

I t used to be somewhat difficult to get a phone number. First you had to have an address, and then you needed someone to come in and physically install the line. Now, however, all you need is a Google Voice account and access to a computer with Internet. The number you get from Google will be yours and can go wherever you and your practice go. It can remain the "face" of your practice going forward. The reason this is step four, rather than a later step, is because patients and clients reach you by phone. If they can call you then they can come to see you, and ultimately, you can get paid. No phone, no money. It is that simple.

So why get a phone before the office, you say? For one thing, the phone is cheap, and an office with furniture, equipment, and staffing is expensive. If you get a phone number and immediately start to book patients or clients, you'll have to find an office quickly; but at least you'll know you may have a fighting chance of paying your rent and other expenses. If, on the other hand, you get the phone number and it never rings, then you can take your time looking for the right office situation. Alternatively you can interpret the lack of phone activity as a sign that perhaps your referral network is not so loyal to you or that your former patients/clients are really not that enamored of you and that they plan to stay put with the practice that canned you only a few days prior. I just think that this is a cheap easy way to get a rough indicator on whether or not you will take only a few or many of your prior patients/clients with you. No doubt this might be a bitter pill for you to swallow; the fact that you were not considered indispensable by your patients or referral network, but the pill is best swallowed before you commit to the seven-year lease and the expensive office equipment. Get the number and hand it out. If you like the response, proceed to step five. Otherwise reconsider your options.

# STEP 5:

# GET AN ANSWERING SERVICE

⸺⸺•◦•⸺⸺

No one was more anti-answering service than I was in the first edition of *Suddenly Solo*. So I surprised even myself when I placed "Get an answering service" as step five. But here is my rationale—answering the phone is critical to your success, and it needs to be done twenty-four seven. Only you can't be the one to do it. It is just physically impossible and wildly impractical. You will be too busy with other things or unavailable when the call comes in or simply not in the mood to take the call. Perhaps you don't like talking on the phone, or maybe your phone voice stinks and you come across poorly on the phone. But the point is that the phone must be answered twenty-four seven.

Oh, voice mail you say? Forget about it! While voice mail may be okay for your established patients who want to get test results, or for a patient who wants to fly in under the radar to cancel an appointment, it is completely unacceptable for any patient or any client, new or even established, who wants to make an appointment to be seen. Unless you are the only game in town—which you are not—or unless you are so busy already—which you are not—then you need those phones manned twenty-four seven by live people. Otherwise the person will just go right down the list to the next doctor. I am sorry, are you not feeling special? Well, it is true. You are not special. Get used to it and move on.

All answering services are not created equal. Many, if not most, answer the phone in a generic sort of way: "Hello, doctor's service" or even worse, "Service." Any new patient who hears this will hang up immediately. These types of services are cheap, but they are not much better than voice mail. The best types of services are ones that function as an extension of your office, like they are your employees. You give them a script and they follow it. They can book appointments and answer questions about the practice. You just have to take the time to develop scripts that pertain to a number of possible call scenarios, and the call service personnel will follow the scripts with a courteous, non-rushed, friendly voice. Your patients and referring doctors will be amazed with how fast you landed on your feet and will be impressed with you. Your practice will be headed in the right direction.

A call center that offers this level of service does not come cheap. They charge by the minute for the calls, and monthly bills can easily exceed $1,000. Of course, if the phone does not ring, you pay nothing, and if the phone rings nonstop with people wanting to come and see you, then your practice is likely to do quite well. If you are willing to spend the time and money to find a call center such as this, train them and pay them appropriately, then proceed to step six. If not, then reconsider your dedication to your solo practice.

# STEP 6:

# GET A WEBSITE

W hen I first went out on my own in 2006, I knew nothing about the web. I did not know a website from a blog from a hole in the wall. I knew nothing about search engines or what a domain name meant. HTML? Couldn't even spell it. Java? No thanks. I prefer Diet Coke. I was using the web at the time for things like e-mail and shopping. Social networking was still in its infancy, and Facebook had not yet been born. I could not build a website to save my life, even with the self-serve website building sites, and professional services were too costly.

I had heard of blogs during the Bush-Kerry presidential campaign, but I had only a vague notion of what a blog was. Why the hell would anyone want to write inane stuff online? What purpose could that possibly serve? But my friend, Steve, a successful Internet 1.0 entrepreneur, told me to just do it. Write anything. Did not matter. He set me up with a blog linked to one of his sites, and my first post went something like this: "Dr. Schoor, male infertility specialist, is now located in Smithtown and can be reached at 631-326-6035." One week later, a patient I had seen several years earlier called my former practice looking for me. He said he did not know where I was, so he looked me up. He Googled "Dr. Schoor male infertility specialist" and immediately got my blog post. He called me, came to the office, and ultimately booked a vasectomy reversal, the proceeds of which funded my first month of operations. Oh, so that is why some blog. Go no!

Getting a website is now very easy and can be DIY'd in about fifteen minutes for free. Your website can be one page long. It can be a blog page or even a Facebook page. Essentially the site needs your name, your phone number (see above), and what you do. You can list your hours—if you have them—and your location—if you have that yet—but at the beginning, it only needs to have your name, phone number, and specialty.

If you feel like getting frisky and think you can build your own site, do it. You can! It is actually pretty simple. Just keep in mind that 4 things matter most for a website: it must have good content, have fast loading webpages, the pages must be uniformly viewable on all the major browser types (IE, Mozilla, Chrome, & Safari) and the site must, must, must be mobile device friendly. Beautifully designed sites with flash video and wonderful graphics may look good, but not only is this unnecessary, flash and graphics can be slow to load and not mobile device friendly. Put your efforts instead into unique content on a hosting platform like Blogger or Wordpress (or the myriad others) that are free and work well on mobile devices and across all browser-types.

How do you get content? You write it yourself. No one knows your specialty better than you and no one else other than you can create content that will be perfect for your site. Want to really be awesome? Try this: produce some videos, host them to YouTube and link the videos to your site. Videos are a great way to get a message across to potential clients, are easy and cheap to produce. Good videos, in my humble opinion, must have 3 elements: good light quality, good sound quality, concise content. If you can't do a video with all 3 elements, don't do one at all.

I just have one more thing to say about content. I think—and this is my view so take it or leave it—that the best content focuses on the needs of the reader, ie the client or prospective patient, rather than the writer—you. I know that you need patients or clients but having content that simply tells people how great you are will not work to attract a single new client. Do not be self-serving and think of content as an advertisement. The best way to attract business is to try to be a part of the solution to another person's problem. Give away your information and knowledge for free. Yep. Free. Then the clients will call.

Still lost? Okay, do this:
1.  Go to Google
2.  Google the word Blogger
3.  Follow instructions to start your own blog
4.  Customize blog by following instructions
5.  Create content

Still confused? Rethink your plan to go solo.

# STEP 7:

# MARKET, MARKET, MARKET.

---

New business will be the life's blood of your fledgling practice, so you best learn how to attract new patients or clients and keep established ones happy—not just returning to your practice, but referring their loved ones to you as well. You must learn to market. It is not enough to be good at what you do. You must learn from where your business comes and to market yourself. In medical practice, patients come from four places: insurance lists, professional referrals, word-of-mouth referrals, and the Internet, and the relative proportions will vary from practice to practice, by specialty, and by geographic location. The same is true for any type of professional service business, except for the insurance referral listings.

Marketing can be divided into two categories: internal and external marketing. Internal marketing is multifaceted. An internal marketing strategy might involve giving in-office seminars to your own patients or sending a letter to your patients about something you learned at a recent conference you attended. Sending a newsletter to your own patients is internal marketing. But internal marketing is so much more than the techniques just mentioned. Internal marketing is also whether or not you return calls promptly and how well you deal with prescription refills, in the case of a health care provider. Internal marketing can be how clean your office is, how friendly the staff is, whether or not you run on time, and if you always have room to "squeeze" someone who wants to be seen into the schedule. Basically, if external marketing is how well you talk the talk, internal marketing is how well you walk the walk. Understand? External marketing can get new patients in the front door, or get a new doctor to throw you a bone, but internal marketing makes your practice thrive; makes it soar. Internal marketing increases word-of-mouth business and repeat referrals. Plus, effective internal marketing means you are a good doctor, a good businessperson. Happy clients recommend friends and family. Unhappy patients dissuade friends, family, acquaintances, and strangers—whoever will listen.

External marketing includes, but is in no way limited to, advertising. External marketing can be, but need not be, expensive. There are many strategies that you can use to promote your practice. Some people advertise in the newspaper, some on radio, some both.

You may wish to hire a practice rep that tries to drum up business for you by going door-to-door on your behalf or you may wish to go door-to-door yourself. You can do "lunch and learns," newsletters, e-mail campaigns, direct mail, Facebook, brochures and on and on. The options are limitless, but so can be the cost.

Many firms exist—and they will come out of the woodwork in the opening weeks of your practice—that specialize in marketing for any industry.

*"Accounting? Sure, we are the leading firm. Oh, medical you said? Sorry, yeah, no one better than us!"*

Should you use one of these firms? Well, that depends, really. Not all marketing firms are created equal, and many firms claim to specialize in medical marketing but actually don't. In addition, some medical marketing firms that appear "big" actually outsource most of their operations—copywriting, search marketing, design, and more—to independent contractors, and not all of those contractors are good. So my advice is to learn the techniques yourself. They are really not that challenging. I actually attended several seminars on marketing techniques that helped me tremendously. I don't actually have anything against the professional marketers, and I have even used some pretty good firms to help me on certain projects, but I do think that when you are an absolute marketing novice, an unscrupulous firm will oversell you on services that you don't need and that won't help.

Before you decide to jump into the wonderful world of external marketing, I recommend that you read up on it and even take some courses. Contact me if you want to know more of what I did.

Having said all that, one strategy does deserve some mention here and now: **Adwords**. Adwords are the banner ads you see on the top and side of the page when you do a Google search for something. You can learn to set up an Adwords campaign and get it functioning in under an hour. The pros can do it, perhaps, in less time, but they can't do it better than you. Trust me on this one. It is actually pretty easy—certainly easier than running your own practice. Google has many tutorials to help you get started, and like anything else, the more you do it, the better you will get at it. Google also has online tools—free tools—that you can use to determine which keyword phrases people use in their searches, which ads get the most clicks, and where these clicks come from. The pros claim they have access to these tools because they are pros, but that is not true. You have equal access to the very same tools. Try it out.

If you don't think you have the gumption to be a good self-promoter and marketer, or that you lack the skill set to get an Adwords account up and running, then you may wish to reconsider your plan to go solo. Otherwise proceed to the next step.

# STEP 8:

# GET A BANK ACCOUNT

---·◦•◦·---

T his is an easy step, but even here mistakes can cost you. You may want to have the bank account be a business one rather than a personal/consumer one. In order to do this, you'll need a tax identification number, a TIN. A TIN is a social security number for a business. In order to get a TIN, you need a corporation; hence step three.

Why can't you just use a personal bank account? You can, but there are some advantages to having a business account. You will want to keep the business money separate from the personal money for tax reasons, but also for liability reasons. If a creditor goes after your business, as long as your personal assets remain separate from the business assets, your liability exposure will be limited. Or if a disgruntled employee sues you for wrongful termination, your business money is at risk but not your personal assets. This separation of corporate and private assets is called a corporate veil, and it is best not to pierce the veil.

On the other hand, personal bank accounts have some advantages over business accounts. The US Congress in recent years has passed a series of banking consumer protection laws that only apply to individuals, rather than businesses. So if you have a business account and business credit cards, you lack the protection that is afforded by law to individuals. Such protections include fraudulent purchase protection and protection against excessive late fee charges, among others. So as you can see, what type of bank account to open is a trade-off between liability protection and consumer protection. Only you can make the decision.

Once you have decided what to do, then proceed to step nine.

# STEP 9:

# UPDATE WITH INSURANCE CARRIERS

———◆◆◆———

This step really just applies to health professionals, so if you are not in the health field, skip to the next section. Otherwise read on.

Now this may seem like an easy step, but it is not. I don't know if the carriers do this intentionally or not, but a mere change of address can delay payments for months. I can't stress enough that this process must be approached carefully, methodically, and deliberately. For this, I recommend hiring a professional who has done this before, and many times.

If you do decide to do it on your own, here is what you must be prepared to do. You will need to contact the provider-relations rep from each and every carrier with which you contract. You will need to complete form after form after form, update your resume, and give the insurance carrier everything they need many times over. The insurance carriers have no incentive to make things easy for you, and they will neglect to follow through on anything and everything. To counter this, you will need to be diligent and meticulous with your record keeping. Every time you speak to a rep from an insurance company or Medicare, take a name and ask for a reference number of the conversation and record it. If this sounds like a very laborious and unpleasant process, it is.

Here is one more thing to keep in mind. If you want any checks to come to your new practice rather than to your old employers, then you must be prepared to delay submitting claims until you are certain that the insurance carrier has completed the change of address process.

Still good? Then proceed to the next step.

# STEP 10:

# GET A CREDIT CARD PROCESSOR

———— ◆◆◆ ————

It took me a while to come to see the value in accepting credit card payments. After all, I thought, why should I give up another 2-3 percent when I already have such high overhead? But people no longer walk around with cash or checks, and if you don't accept credit card payments, you have to send bills in the mail and wait for people to pay you. Let me tell you— once someone leaves the office, your chance of being paid drops dramatically. Even if they do pay you, the patient might take thirty, sixty, or even ninety days to do it, yet your bills come due every thirty days.

One other thing—accept Visa, MasterCard, and American Express. Without fail, the one you don't accept will be the only card the patient or client has in the wallet at the time of service. Never give someone a reason to delay paying you. Instead make it easy to pay. AMEX? Fine. Diner's Club? Sure. PayPal? Why the hell not?

So why did I choose this step now, as step ten? Because you may start seeing clients any day now, and you will need to start to collect money; even if it is only copays, in the case of a doctor. But don't kid yourself; not only do the copays add up to real money, but the copays are often more than what the insurance companies disburse to you. So when someone comes to see you, collect the payment up front, either by cash or credit card (not personal check).

How does one actually go about obtaining a credit card processor? Very easily. You just need to apply for a merchant account with a bank. If you don't think you can figure this out on your own, then perhaps you are not ready to open your own practice. If you can figure it out, then proceed to the next step.

# STEP 11:

# GET AN EMR
## (INVEST IN INFORMATION TECHNOLOGY)

---

No business today can function well without utilizing modern and efficient information technology. Can you imagine paying an accountant who did not have accounting software to do your tax services? Of course not. If you plan to open your own professional services business, you must embrace information technology and its costs. The medical field is no different in this capacity, except that doctors have been slow to adopt information technology. However, like it or not, EMR technology has arrived and is here to stay[2]. And this is a good thing. The EMR is your friend. A good EMR is like an employee, really; only one who is never sick and is always

---

2  *I use EMR and EHR interchangeably, but there is a difference. EMRs are basically medical charts in digital format. EHRs include that, plus everything else that is needed to run a complex health organization. What you want is an EHR.

ready to do the job you ask of it. EMRs will help you function with more efficiency and with fewer mistakes and less aggravation. You will have fewer pharmacy-related issues and pharmacy callbacks. You will be able to disposition the results of inbound labs and radiology studies quickly and with little effort. Abnormal lab results will never get lost in the ether only to come back to bite you in the behind later. You will never have to search for a patient chart. With regard to billing, EMRs make billing very simple. A good one will automatically queue the encounter for your biller to examine, scrub (make sure that everything is linked and correct so the claim will not be rejected on technical terms) and then forward to the clearinghouse[3]. A good EMR will also allow you to run reports on virtually anything, like how many prescriptions you write for drug X, how many new patients you saw last month, and how many people were sent for CT scans in the last nine days.

The EMR you get should be robust and capable of growing with the practice. While you don't want to go bankrupt paying for the system, you never want to outgrow it either. Personally I recommend combined EMR and PM (practice management) solutions, though

---

3 ** What is a clearinghouse? Clearinghouses receive your claims prior to passing them onto the individual insurance carriers. They are middlemen, and they extract a fee coming and going. You can avoid paying clearinghouse fees by submitting claims on paper—which I do not recommend.

not everyone agrees with me. The system should have charting features, a scheduler, robust reporting capabilities, and be CCHIT certified. The company that sells you the EMR must be able to provide twenty-four seven support and ought to be a reputable firm. You'd be surprised to learn that many an EMR company has gone belly-up. In some of these situations, the doctors completely lost access to all of their patients' medical records and billing data. A few practices even went out of business as a result.

If you don't see the usefulness of an EMR or simply refuse to use one, then please reconsider your plan to go solo. Otherwise proceed to the next step.

# STEP 12:

# FIND OFFICE SPACE

———

Iknow, I know. Having this step last seems totally bonkers and it still amazes me that this is the final step in the process, rather than the first. In fact, when I opened up my own office in 2006, this was the first step I took. Moreover, everyone who has ever contacted me regarding their own suddenly solo experiences have told me that the first item on their own to-do lists was to find office space. In the first edition of *Suddenly Solo*, I even listed "find office space" at the top of the must-do list. This seems obvious, and of course it is, because you really can't see patients or clients in Starbucks or the public library. But now, after close to seven years of planning new ventures and helping others achieve their goals, I have become convinced that office space must be the last step in the process. Why? All other steps can be undone and modified easily and without much cost to you. Office space, on the other hand, can be like herpes—you're stuck with it. If after you have completed the prior eleven steps and your phone is ringing and you have demand for your services, you can then lease or sublease an office. On the other hand, if the phone never rings, perhaps you should rethink the plan for the multiyear lease and go for a month-to-month lease (or get a job). Are you beginning to see my rationale?

Now what type of office space you acquire at this step can really impact your future ability to make money. When it comes to office space, you must consider many things: square footage, location, parking, layout, build out, neighbors, terms of lease, and so forth.

Your ideal office should be in a location that prospective patients can get to easily. In a suburban location this means in in a high visibility complex with ample parking. If you intend to practice in a large pedestrian city, then pick an office in proximity to public transportation. The physical office should be large enough to see as many patients per hour as possible with comfort. It should have a front office/reception area and a separate exit area. The office should also have a separate back-office area for functions like billing and collection and, in general fighting like a banshee for your money. Ideally the office will not require much of a build-out. What is a build-out? Just like it sounds: constructing walls, plumbing, cabinetry, carpeting, and so on for the office. Build-outs can costs tens to hundreds of thousands of dollars, even millions of dollars. So if you find an office that can work without a major build-out, jump on it. I know of a dentist that spent over a million on his new office-mahogany walls and cabinets, plush carpets, fine art; the works. It looked amazing but it sunk not just his practice but his personal finances as well. Just beware.

The rent ought to be reasonable and affordable. Notice I did not say cheap. I said reasonable. Rent is based on all the above factors plus a host of others. Don't base your decision entirely on the dollar amount of the rent. For example, if you want to be a Park Avenue plastic surgeon, it helps to have an office on Park Avenue, rather than Jackson Avenue. Having an office that is too small will cost you as well in terms of bottlenecks and decreased efficiency.

At first, consider subleasing from another doctor, either of a different specialty or even your own (if you can). This is a great way to drastically reduce costs. You won't need to buy furniture or standard medical equipment. Plus, with current telephone technology, you can have your own virtual office complete with staffing, so you won't even need to rely on your landlord's receptionist to book patients. I think this is great way, though I did not do it this way. Why? I made a mistake. But in my defense, I found the perfect office that needed no build out. It was walk-in ready. Every other office space I looked at was a disaster area. Al I was okay financially, so I could afford the rent. Even so, if I had to do it all again, I would find a doctor, or several doctors, and sublease from them a few sessions per week. Only after I had a bona fide and reliable patient following would I take a lease on an office of my own and take on those costs.

Finally how does one go about finding office space? There are several ways to do it. You can hire an agent, and the agent does the grunt work on your behalf. Just keep in mind that the agent is typically paid by, and thus works for, the landlord, not you, so their incentives might not match up with yours. In addition, the agent's fee is based on the value of the lease, so if you are looking for an inexpensive, month-to-month or nonstandard type of deal, an agent might not even wish to work on your behalf.

So that leaves us with option number two: walking around. This is not so bad, if you have the time to do it. By driving from office park to office park, you will see signs that say something like, "call xxx-yyyy for office space availability." With your cell phone, you simply call xxx-yyyy and go from there. It is that simple, really.

But what if you don't have the time to drive around? No problem. Turn to the web, option number three. Personally I like Craigslist.com, and have had success in the past using it to find available subleases. Any agent or landlord worth anything will post listings to Craigslist. Plus, you can post that you are looking for space, and ultimately, someone will contact you. There are also other real estate listing services on the web that you can Google, but Craigslist.com is a good place to start.

Now for option four: word of mouth. Like any form of referral, word of mouth from a trusted source to another trusted source is the best. In this case, you would simply ask colleagues, pharmaceutical reps, your medical equipment vendor—whomever—if they know of anyone looking to sublease some space.

Think you can handle this? Great. If not, then re-think your plan to go solo. Otherwise proceed.

# ARE YOU READY?

————————

While there is no way to really be 100 percent prepared to be on your own, solo, and responsible for your own destiny, if you go through the twelve-step process I have described, you will be ready when the time comes. I know this based on my own experience, and through the shared experiences of many other people just like you. You do not have to reinvent the wheel. Just do these twelve steps. After you complete all twelve steps—really and truly complete them rather than just read about them—all that remains for you to do is to find a biller, see patients, and start billing. You will have done the rest.

See, you are ready. Congratulations.

One last thing: when can you start the twelve steps? I know I devoted a section to this already, but it is worth mentioning again here. You can start the process now. You can start if you are still employed. You can start even if you are happily employed. You can start if you are a resident or a new associate with a group. You can even start if you are an academic physician looking to build your brand.

Of course, you need to start if you already have been sacked.

# IF I COULD DO IT ALL AGAIN: THE TURNKEY WIRELESS OFFICE OF TWENTY-FIRST CENTURY.

———••———

If I were to do it again, I think I would do it this way: I would find a doctor and rent a room from him once or twice per week. The lease would be short-term, month-to-month, and be for the use of the room, some parking, and some medical equipment like gauze pads and Band-Aids—nothing else.

My IT infrastructure would consist of a laptop computer, a wireless hotspot (4G), a network portable printer, and a web-based EMR—a free one like Practice Fusion.

My only expensive medical device would be a portable ultrasound unit with color flow and Doppler and two probes (can't live without it).

For phones, I would use a cellphone and an answering service, like the one mentioned in step five. Patients could communicate with me by phone (discouraged) or by secure online messaging via a service, such as www.Twistle.com (encouraged).

If I could make my overhead without contracting with insurance companies, I would do so from day one. If non-par was not possible, I would outsource billing in the beginning, with the ultimate goal of taking it in-house.

All appointment requests would be handled online or over the phone.

I would collect all payments, such as copays and cash pay/self-pay patients, using a credit card processor attached to a smartphone.

I would determine what aspect of practice I enjoyed the most and what I was best at (hopefully they would be the same), and would actively promote that aspect of my practice from the onset. All marketing activities would stay focused and on-target for this area of specialty.

I would have a website from day one and promote using Adwords from day one.

Operationally, the practice would function something like this:

- Prospective patients would either find me online, by word of mouth or through professional referral and call. The phone would be answered immediately, twenty-four seven. The call center would take all information and I would confirm. Modest appointment fee would be taken ahead of time by credit card and stored via third party processor (EasyPay Solutions Inc., Exchange EDI Inc., and more. [4*]). If he/she no-shows, the no-show fee is charged. Patient is made aware of this ahead of time. Insurance eligibility (if applicable) verified ahead of time by billing agency.
- I would have no paper forms other than HIPAA and ABN. These forms get scanned into system. I collect ID and insurance card (if applicable) and collect copay amount in room with patient using mobile CC processor. No checks. Cash is fine. I then perform my medical services. Labs are ordered via EMR interface, and all prescriptions either e-prescribed or printed by my portable network printer.
- I exit patient and next patient is then roomed.
- Thirty minutes for new patients.
- Fifteen for established.

---

4  [*] I have no financial interest with either of these companies.

- Patients that come late may or may not be accommodated, depending on schedule and no-shows.

Total overhead for this type of practice:
- Liability insurance-fixed
- Rent-fixed
- Answering service-variable
- EMR-free
- Cellphone and hotspot ~$200 per month
- CC fees-variable, 2-3 percent
- Billing service—variable, 5-8 percent
- Marketing—variable, ~3-5 percent of gross revenue
- Incorporation ~$1,000 as a one-time cost
- Licensing ~$500 per two years, varies per state
- DEA ~$750 per three years

This is a good way to start. It will allow you to keep overhead rock bottom until you can afford to hire a staff, get a bigger office, take on equipment leases, and so forth.

# CONCLUSION

———— ••• ————

I love solo, independent practice. I thrive on it, actually—the constant change, the challenge of bringing in new business, the control, the fact that the practice is mine and mine alone, and the dream of growth. But solo practice is not for everybody. If after reading this book you realize that solo practice is not for you—you lack the financial support, the marketing savvy, the attention to detail, the timeline—then get a job. There is absolutely nothing wrong with that. Most people in the world want jobs and a steady paycheck, nothing more. There is no reason that you cannot find satisfaction via professional and personal growth, yet still be an employed, salaried physician. The key is to find the right employer, the right job, and to develop a different type of mind-set. The great thing about medicine is that it can be both a job and a career. Having said that, for many of us, only solo independent practice can provide us with the professional and personal happiness that we want. If I am describing you, and you believe that you can get through all twelve steps, then proceed to step thirteen and take the plunge.

## CONCLUSION

I wish you good luck in your endeavors, no matter what you decide. Please drop me a line and let me know how it is going: rich@drschoor.com.

The End

# APPENDIX 1:

------◦◦◦------

*What is an RVU?*

All medical procedures are assigned relative value units, RVUs. Medicare assigns the number of RVUs to an individual procedure. For example, a follow-up visit for an established patient may have only one RVU assigned to it, while a coronary angiogram might be worth one thousand RVUs. RVUs in and of themselves have no financial value but Medicare—and by extension some private payers—determine reimbursements based on RVUs. RVUs can also be used to see how hard a doctor is working and as such his/her compensation can be tied to the number of RVUs they generate each year. You may be able to see already how the system can be gamed. A doctor who sits all day doing lithotripsies (a high RVU/low effort kidney stone procedure) will generate ten times the RVUs of the doctor who sees fifty patients a day in the office and the hospital. As a result, some doctors seem to almost forget their Hippocratic oaths as they compete with themselves and amongst each other to maximize RVU generation. This is a very unpleasant—yet very common—way to be a doctor. Most hospital/corporate physician-employee arrangements are based in some way on RVU generation.

# APPENDIX 2:

Sample Rough and Dirty Business Plan

1. Office Space
    a. Use a broker
    b. Drive around the office parks
    c. Craigslist
    d. Talk to colleagues about a sublease
2. Furniture
    a. Garage sales
    b. Office Max
    c. Buy versus rent
3. Phones
    a. How many?
    b. Virtual systems

    c. Cell phones only

4. Computers—but how many?

    a. Laptop for me

    b. Receptionist computer

    c. Draw office map

5. Phone number

6. Exam Tables

7. Medical Supplies

    a. Contact PSS or Schein

    b. Talk to office managers from other practices

8. Insurance (but what type?)

    a. Talk to broker

    b. Ask other doctors/managers

9. Financing

    a. Family

    b. Savings

    c. Loans versus leasing versus line of credit

10. Patients

    a. Go door-to-door begging

    b. Adwords

    c. Ad in local paper

    d. Hire marketing rep

11. Marketing

    a. Need knowledge

        i. Read books

        ii. Conference

        iii. Ask doctors, other small business

12. Call coverage

13. Answering service

14. Hospital privileges

    a. Drive to local hospital

    b. Complete application myself

    c. Hire consultant

15. Credentialing

    a. Call reps

    b. Hire consultant

    c. Talk to docs/managers

16. Staff

    a. Ad on Craigslist

    b. Call the local MA schools

    c. Help wanted ad

17. Payroll service

    a. Talk to my accountant

    b. Contact ADP, Paychex

# APPENDIX 3:

---

*Sample Phone Scenarios and Scripts*

Patient wants appointment:

> Good (morning/afternoon/evening) thank you for calling (Medical Practice Name). This is (name) speaking. How may I help you?

> That is no problem. Do you have any preferences for when you would like to be seen?

> Our hours are (list hours). Do any of these times work for you?

> Is this an emergency or do you need to be seen today?

> Okay, we just need some basic information now. May we have your name?

> Many of our patients have the same name. So we don't get confused, may we have your date

of birth? Great. Okay, what is the best number for us to reach you? Great.

How did you learn about our practice?

Someone from the office will call you back to confirm the appointment.

Is there anything else we can assist you with today?

Patient wants to cancel appointment:
> Good (morning/afternoon/evening) thank you for calling (Medical Practice Name). This is (name) speaking. How may I help you?
>
> That is no problem. May I ask the reason for the cancellation? Would you like to reschedule the appointment now?
>
> Okay, we will pass that along to the office. Thank you for letting us know, and if there is anything else you need from us do not hesitate to contact us.

Patient wants test results:
> Good (morning/afternoon/evening) thank you for calling (Medical Practice Name). This is (name) speaking. How may I help you?

That is no problem.

Many of our patients have the same name. So we don't get confused may we have your date of birth? Great. Okay, what is the best number for us to reach you? Great.

What test result are you looking for?

Okay, someone from the office will contact you by the end of the day today. Is that okay? Or do you need to be contacted sooner?

Okay, I will pass that along to the office, and thank you for calling. If you do not hear back from someone in what you consider to be a timely fashion, please call us back.

Patient inquiry about practice (do you take such and such insurance, address, and so forth.):

> Good (morning/afternoon/evening) thank you for calling (Medical Practice Name). This is (name) speaking. How may I help you?

> I will be happy to help you with that. Did you know that most information about the practice can be found on our website, like insurance participation, office hours, address, services provided? Have you seen our website?

Doctor/ER/Hospital/Patient with emergency calls to talk to doctor:

> Good (morning/afternoon/evening) thank you for calling (Medical Practice Name). This is (name) speaking. How may I help you?
>
> That is no problem.
>
> Would you like me to page him/her, or if you can hold, I can get the doctor on the phone right now?

Sales call:

> Good (morning/afternoon/evening) thank you for calling (Medical Practice Name). This is (name) speaking. How may I help you?
>
> Go to hell (alternatively, "Eat shit and die."

# APPENDIX 4:

———— ••• ————

*Pitfalls of Sublease Arrangements That You Must Avoid*

Beware of subleasing from primary care doctors who offer to help build your practice through patient referrals. These guys can be poison. Here is how the business model works. He/she has a very busy primary care practice and a very large office. To augment income, the doctors sublease space to specialists, medical imaging companies, and diagnostic testing companies. The tenants pay rent to the doctor, who in turn refers their patients to the tenants for consults or testing. The arrangement can be legit as long as the following criteria are met: referrals must be medically necessary and the lease states that the rent is only for square footage, equipment staffing, parking area, and that the rent cannot change until a period of one year has transpired. What is not legit is to pay for referrals. This is called a kickback scheme, and you go to jail for this. Even so, some people who enter these types of arrangements have an unspoken agreement about the true nature of the relationship: you rent from me, I give you patients. In many cases, the doctor doing the leasing even offers to maintain your patients' charts. Isn't that generous! What happens, though, is that initially the doctor feeds you with lots of referrals, then he/she finds some novel way to extract more money from you. When you refuse, the referrals dry up. When you go to leave, the doctor has control of your patients' charts. Not good. Stay away from this at all costs.

The better way to sublease is to make it clear from the get-go that you just need the physical space and perhaps some staffing/equipment, but nothing else. You will take care of how you get your patients and how and where you keep the charts (think EMR). When the doctor thinks he owns you, you tell him to get lost and you walk away. No biggie. The key is to be beholden to yourself only—well, maybe your spouse as well.

# APPENDIX 5:

———— ••• ————

*To take insurance or not to take insurance; that is the question.*

While dealing with insurance companies complicates the business of medicine and makes it more expensive (even though managed care was supposed to drive costs down!), this fact should not deter you from participating with managed care contracts. Instead you must take a rational approach that factors in local market forces and out-of-network rates versus in-network rates for your specialty in your community. This is no easy task.

The decision regarding whether or not to participate with insurance plans depends on a number of factors: specialty, geographic location, and the degree of competition within your market. Specialties like general surgery & orthopedics have a high percentage of emergency care that, by law, insurance companies must pay for— regardless of whether or not the doctor is in-network or out-of-network. A specialty such as urology—my specialty—has very little emergency care. This is one reason why I picked urology as my specialty. However, this characteristic makes it more difficult for me to go out-of- network and get higher rates with the insurance carriers. A family practice doctor may decide that he or she will get such low rates from insurance carriers that it makes sense to not bother contracting with them in the first place. In this type of case, the family practice doctor would just charge reasonable fees that his or her community could afford, or the doctor can choose a concierge-type model.

Geographic location matters as well. If you plan to practice in a saturated marketplace, like NY metro or south Florida, then you may find yourself at too much of a competitive disadvantage if you choose to be out-of-network. In another community which has very few of your type of doctor, you may be able to remain out-of-network and do well.

The decision to participate or not with insurance contracts is not a personal one. It is based on simple mathematics. Can you do better financially by going par or non-par? It is really that simple. The actual analyses by which you come to that determination can be very complicated, but the decision itself, once the determination is made, is simple.

Just one more thing: insurance companies have been lobbying state legislators to limit the excessive out-of-network fees that many doctors charge. In a growing number of states, in-network and out-of-network fee disparities have been minimized. In other words, in or out, you get paid the same. The only difference is that you get paid faster in-network.

So you decide.

# APPENDIX 6:

*Four Strategies to Turbocharge Your Start-Up Practice*

## 1: Take Over A Struggling Practice

Acquiring a struggling practice or that of an aging or retiring doctor can be a great way to go. By doing this, you pick up a practice full of patients—presumably paying ones—and then bring your technology and energy into the practice to revitalize it. In the past, these practices were worth hundreds of thousands of dollars, but not anymore. In the present era, most medical practices are worth very little. Specialty practices are worth even less than primary care practices. The trick is to find one of these practices to take over.

Once the practice is acquired, you can employ the doctor for a period of time, see the patients yourself at that location, have the patients travel to your location, hire a physician assistant or nurse practitioner to see the patients at that location or yours, or any combination of the above. Ideally the practice would have several thousand *active* patients, as these are the only patients of any value to you.

The only major problem you may face is what to do with the morass of paper records that you acquire. Do you scan them all into a digital format or leave them alone? Scanning can become very expensive, so if you plan to do this, take it out of the purchase price of the practice. Charts greater than seven years old (ten years for Medicare) can and should be destroyed.[5*] The remaining charts can be archived in a storage facility for a lot less than the cost of scanning. Personally I would leave most legacy charts on paper, unscanned, and prospectively enter any new information into my EHR as I saw the patient. Any pertinent data from the legacy chart could be scanned into my new system, of course.

## 2: Join an IPA

Independent Physician Associations (IPAs) are hybrids between the multispecialty groups and totally independent practices. In a multispecialty group, the doctors are employees of the group (even if they are partners as well), and the group has a single corporate structure. In an IPA, each independent doctor/doctor

5   [*] Rules for when you can destroy a chart vary from state to state. Medicare and commercial insurance plans also have their own rules. Medicaid's rules are different from Medicare's. Prior to destroying a medical record, consult with a health law attorney.

group maintains 100 percent of their independence, corporate structure, and tax identification number. A membership in the IPA gets you some of the advantages of being in a larger group, such as group purchasing power, assistance with managed care contract negotiation, legal and business services, and others, yet it allows you to remain completely independent. In some of these IPAs, doctors may have a vested interest in referring to other member doctors. Even if they don't have such an interest, membership allows you to go to the IPA meetings where you can meet the other doctors and press the flesh. In the current era of super busy doctors who no longer have the time to hang out in doctors' lounges or have the money to belong to country clubs, membership in an IPA might be the best way to initiate a more personal relationship with potential referring doctors.

3: Join an ACO

ACOs—Accountable Care Organizations—are the newest iteration of the shared savings-shared risk model of health care delivery and financing. In an ACO model, Medicare (or the private payer) determines a benchmark cost for care to a certain community and encourages the organization—the ACO—to deliver care to that community below the benchmark cost. If the ACO accomplishes the goal, then it gets a percentage of the savings returned to it in the form of a bonus payment. If it does not meet the goal, it does not get the money.[6]* Member doctors of an ACO are under pressure to deliver high quality care at less cost and *all* the doctors/members of an ACO must be on the same page and be indoctrinated into the same mantra of high quality care over high quantity care in order to maximize the chance of getting the bonus payment. As such, these doctors have a very strong incentive to refer to doctors that share these goals. Therefore, if you are a member of such an ACO and you share their goals, they will refer to you.

Understand?

## 4: Get On Multiple On-Call Schedules

Personally I am not a big fan of this because I don't like taking hospital ER call. However, for many doctors, taking call at one or more hospitals is a great way to get very busy, very fast. This is especially true for specialties like general surgery, orthopedics, cardiology, and gastroenterology, among others. Also, if you can pull off the out-of-network insurance billing thing, you can do really well financially with this type of arrangement.

---

6   * There are 2 types of ACO risk models. In one model, the ACO accepts a lower saving percentage savings but takes no risk if the benchmark is not met. In the other model, the ACO gets more money but risks losing money if costs exceed the benchmarked costs.

Personally I have some issues with this model, but I totally understand why many find it attractive. For one thing, you can make a lot of money doing it. It requires very little knowledge or skills in external marketing and costs you next to nothing—basically just the cost of gas to and from the hospital. Also, once you get the patients from the hospital and you "wow" them and their families with your skills and charm, you can then grow your practice even more through increased word-of-mouth referrals.

Except it just does not work this way. It is extremely difficult to "wow" a patient/family as the on-call doc. The best time to meet patients and their families and establish a positive and trusting relationship with them is by referral from a trusted doctor or family member, not from an ER physician who the patient and family has met only minutes before and during a time of great duress. In a situation like this, the consultant doctor gets zero points for doing a good job, but gets all the blame when there is a complication or when the patient simply does not do well. In these types of situations, you can only win by not losing. One other thing about growing a practice by being the on-call doctor: when you grow it this way you will be stuck with it long after the thrill of it has diminished.

I think there are better ways to build a practice with staying power and intrinsic value.

# RESOURCES

————◆————

Though you may feel like it, you are not alone. Many have stood where you stand now, and have not only done it, they have written about it. I recommend the following:

- The MGMA (Medical Group Management Association)
- The American Urologic Association Practice Managers Network (must be a member of the AUA)
- *Marketing Your Clinical Practice 3rd edition,* Neil Baum and Judith Henkel
- *Think Business!* Owen Dahl
- Health Care Success Strategies (http://www.healthcaresuccess.com/) website, blogs, and CD-ROM
- The public library for any book on marketing and business

Visit my blog site, www.theindependenturologist.com, for information about my webinars, seminars, and coaching offers.